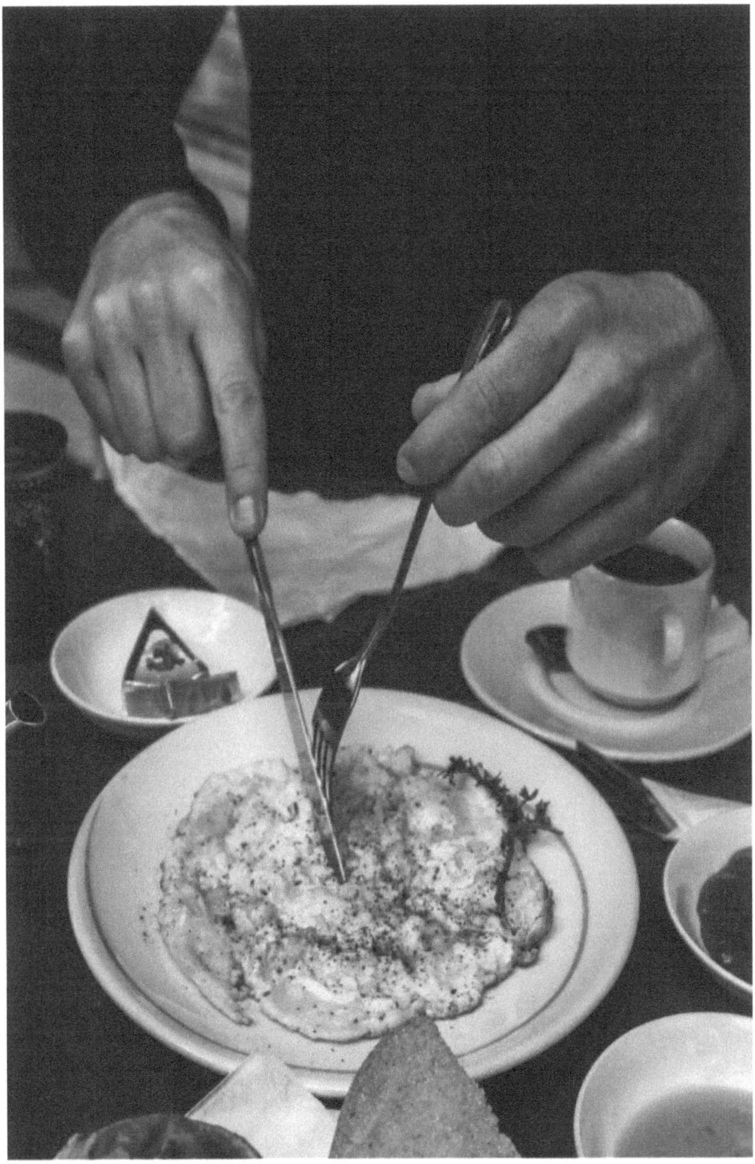

The Ultimate Guide to Losing Weight on the Ketogenic Diet!

Author

Lisa English

My name is Lisa English and my mission is to help anyone I can to lose weight, and chose a healthier lifestyle.

Through my brand and other platforms I will do the best I can to educate and help anyone I can who suffers from health issues related to their diet.

Acknowledgements

How to Lose the Maximum Weight on Keto?

The difference is intermittent fasting!
Two Types of Ketosis
Nutritional Ketosis & Stored Fat-
Burning
Or
Optimal Ketosis!

Here is the difference!

During Nutritional Ketosis, you are burning the foods you eat. After that happens during fasting, you start to burn the actual stored fat in your body. Like your stomach fat! Which is the ultimate goal right?

Blood Ketone Levels

Blood ketones over 3.0 mmol/L, your body is using your stored fat for fuel. You want this while in fat loss mode. The Ketogenic diet is very scientific! You can control these levels by using your Macros (Protein, Fats, and Carbs), exercise & intermittent fasting!

Intermittent fasting was the key to getting fat adapted!

At the beginning, you need more fat to switch from burning glucose to fat. Now once you are in Ketosis you can get deeper into Ketosis by fasting & lowering your fat & protein to get into body fat burning mode. Here is how I determined how many grams of fat & protein I needed to do this.

Protein & Fat (Weight) x .4-4.5 Grams for maximum weight loss Example if you weigh 200 lbs. (200 x .4=80 grams of fat & protein)

Once you stop eating for the day your body then burns the fat you ate first, then when that is gone it then begins to burn your stored fat for fuel. So the longer you fast the more fat comes off and the more the scales move! You must be in Ketosis a while to become adapted! So do not rush it.

I advise starting slow with intermittent fasting. Start with 8 hours. Then try 9, work up each day until you get comfortable. Try 2 times a week if this is more comfortable.

If you feel, any of these symptoms (stop fast and eat!)! You may not be getting enough nutrients! Too many days can lead to adverse symptoms.

Prolonged fasting may cause vitiation of Vata in the body, and may lead to anxiety, fear, nervousness and weakness.

Fasting for a long term may lead to anemia, irregular heartbeat, a weakened immune system and liver or kidney problems.

Fasting to lose weight can also result in vitamin deficiencies from lack of important minerals. You may fall sick and could have other health problems so pay attention to your body.

Types of Intermittent Fasting

(12/12 Fast) Fast/12, Eat/12 (3 Meals) No snacks

16/8 (Most Common) Fast 16/Eat/8 (2 to 3 meals)

18/6. Fast 18/Eat 6 (Usually 2 meals)

20/4. Fast 20/Eat 4 (1 large meal)

I prefer the 12/12, 16/8, or 14/10.

Do not jump into the deep end of the pool at the beginning. Please work up to longer periods. You should not be starving if you are shortening your fasting.

Drink bulletproof coffee no sweetener, lemon water with a dash of salt, or black coffee with a 1/2 t of butter. Bone broth is good too. Whatever curbs your hunger?

Only use sweetener during your eating window make sure you get your veggies, and nutrients. That makes the fasting easier. Especially your last meal of the day.

During & after your weight loss you need to adjust your macros as you go using the same formula!

Maintenance

Average or Maintenance=Weight x 0.5 thru 0.7 grams.

You will not go into Ketoacidosis, unless you have Type 1 diabetes. There are very rare cases for Type 2.

When Ketoacidosis does occur you would immediately know because your Glucose & Ketones would be high!

Normal people the higher your ketones the lower your glucose! I check my ketone levels & glucose together.

Optimal Blood ketone Levels

Between 0.5-1.5 is light nutritional ketosis. You will be getting a good effect on your weight loss, but not in the optimal fat burning zone.

Around 1.5-3 mmol/L is what is called optimal ketosis and is recommended for maximum weight loss.

Values over 3 mmol/L are in the optimal therapeutic zone usually 3.0-5.0 mmolL.

This usually occurs when intermittent fasting. Fasting ketosis is between the ranges of 5.0-10

Anything above 10 is ketoacidosis which usually only occurs in type 1 diabetics.

Most people's blood ketones range 5.0-8.0 for optimal therapeutic ketosis. When Blood ketones are high and glucose numbers are low there is no danger of ketoacidosis.

If your ketones are high and glucose is high then seek medical attention immediately. If ketoacidosis is your concern, and keeping you from trying the ketogenic diet, and you are type 2 diabetic, then purchase a blood ketone meter and check your numbers!

Then that will eliminate any concerns you may have!

Checking Your GKI
What is GKI?

GKI (Glucose Ketone Index) Levels

GKI is the Blood Glucose & Blood Ketone Ratio in your bloodstream

Formula for figuring GKI

Glucose divided by 18 then divided by Blood Ketones

Glucose 86 divided by 18 divided by Ketones 3.6=1.3

Glucose-Ketone Levels

9 & higher means your body has not transitioned into a fat-burning state.

A 6-9 GKI means a low level of ketosis: This is appropriate for those who want to lose weight or maintain optimal health.

A 3-6 GKI means moderate levels of ketosis: This is appropriate for treating metabolic diseases like insulin resistance, Type 2 diabetes, & obesity.

A less than 3 GKI is a high level of ketosis: You are in the intermittent fasting for optimal ketosis Fat Burning Mode!

This is generally the level for treating epilepsy and cancers. You do not have to buy a ketone meter to achieve this!

First thing to do keep your total carbs preferably below 20, but each individual is different. I can go up to 30 and still be deep into ketosis.

I just reached a 12-hour Fast, and I will go until I am hungry. For me this is usually 12-16 hours. I break my fast immediately if I do not feel 100% energized.

I worked up to this slowly. I am utilizing fasting for weight loss. Once I reach my goal weight, I may use fasting 2 to 3 times a week for the health benefits of fasting.

Disclaimer:

This is what works for me. Do what works best for you. Research these facts for yourself. Of course, always consult your doctor.

Website:

Ketohappyeatfatnotcarbs.com

Email Ketohappy@gmail.com

Keto Happy Eat Fat Not Carbs
Facebook Page

https://www.facebook.com/ketohappye
atfatnotcarbs

Facebook Group

https://www.facebook.com/groups/KetoHappy/

I hope you enjoyed this book!

Please leave a review on Amazon, and if this book helps you along in your keto journey!

The End

www.ingramcontent.com/pod-product-compliance
Lightning Source LLC
Chambersburg PA
CBHW031335290526
45784CB00014B/2765